JOINT PAIN NO MORE

Natural Remedy for Joint Pain

By

Dr. Lunar Stone

Copyright © 2023 Dr. Lunar Stone

TABLE OF CONTENTS

INTRODUCTION

Joint pain is a common symptom experienced by people of all ages. It is often characterized by discomfort, swelling, stiffness, and aching sensations in the joints. The joints are the points in the body where two or more bones come together, allowing movement and support. Joint pain can affect any joint in the body, including the knees, hips, shoulders, wrists, and ankles. The causes of joint pain can be attributed to various factors, including medical conditions, injuries, and lifestyle factors.

Joint pain is a common condition that affects millions of people around the world. It can occur in any joint in the body, including the knees, hips, shoulders, and fingers. Joint pain can be caused by a variety of factors, including injury, arthritis, and other medical conditions. The severity of joint pain can range from mild discomfort to excruciating pain that can limit a person's ability to perform daily activities.

Joints are the connecting points of bones in the body. They allow for movement and flexibility. The bones in a joint are covered with a layer of cartilage, which helps to cushion and protect them. The joints are also surrounded by a capsule that contains synovial fluid, which lubricates the joint and helps it move smoothly.

When the joints are healthy, they function properly, and movement is easy and pain-free. However, when the joints are damaged or become inflamed, they can cause pain and discomfort. Joint pain can be acute, meaning it comes on suddenly and is usually short-lived, or chronic, which is a long-term condition that can last for months or even years.

Acute joint pain is usually caused by an injury, such as a sprain or strain. It can also be caused by overuse of a joint, such as in the case of a repetitive motion injury. Chronic joint pain is often associated with conditions such as arthritis, which causes inflammation in the joints.

CHAPTER 1

SYMPTOMS AND CAUSES

Symptoms

The symptoms of joint pain can vary depending on the cause and severity of the condition. Common symptoms of joint pain include:

- Pain or tenderness in the affected joint(s)

- Stiffness or reduced range of motion in the joint(s)

- Swelling or inflammation in the joint(s)

- Warmth or redness in the affected area

- Difficulty using the joint(s)

- Weakness or instability in the joint(s)

- Grinding or popping sensations when using the joint(s)

Joint pain can be mild or severe, and it can occur in one joint or multiple joints at once. Some people may experience joint pain that is constant, while others may only experience pain during certain activities, such as exercise or after prolonged periods of inactivity.

Causes

Medical conditions

1. Arthritis

Arthritis is one of the most common causes of joint pain. It is a group of diseases that cause inflammation and damage to the joints, resulting in pain, stiffness, and swelling. There are many types of arthritis, including osteoarthritis, rheumatoid arthritis, psoriatic arthritis, and gout. Osteoarthritis is the most common type of arthritis and is caused by the wear and tear of the cartilage that cushions the joints. Rheumatoid arthritis is an autoimmune disease that causes the body to attack its own joints, resulting in inflammation and damage.

2. Lupus

Lupus is an autoimmune disease that can cause joint pain, among other symptoms. It occurs when the body's immune system attacks healthy tissues and organs, leading to inflammation and damage. Lupus can affect any part of the body, including the joints, skin, kidneys, and brain.

3. Lyme disease

Lyme disease is a bacterial infection that is transmitted through the bite of an infected tick. It can cause joint pain, among other symptoms. If left untreated, Lyme disease can lead to chronic joint pain, fatigue, and neurological problems.

4. Fibromyalgia

Fibromyalgia is a chronic condition that causes widespread pain, fatigue, and other symptoms. It is characterized by tender points in the body, including the joints. The cause of fibromyalgia is not well understood, but it is believed to be related to changes in the way the brain processes pain signals.

Injuries

1. Sprains and strains

Sprains and strains are common injuries that can cause joint pain. A sprain occurs when a ligament, the tissue that connects bones to each other, is stretched or torn. A strain occurs when a muscle or tendon, the tissue that connects muscles to bones, is stretched or torn. These injuries can occur from a fall, twist, or other physical activity.

2. Fractures

A fracture is a broken bone that can cause joint pain. When a bone is broken, it can affect the surrounding joints, leading to pain, stiffness, and swelling.

3. Dislocations

A dislocation occurs when a bone is forced out of its normal position. It can cause joint pain, swelling, and limited mobility.

Lifestyle factors

1. Overuse

Overuse of the joints can lead to joint pain. This can occur from repetitive motions or activities that put stress on the joints, such as running, jumping,

or lifting heavy objects.

2. Obesity

Obesity can put extra stress on the joints, leading

to joint pain. It can also increase the risk of

developing osteoarthritis, a common type of

arthritis.

3. Lack of exercise

Lack of exercise can lead to joint pain, as it can

cause the muscles and ligaments around the joints

to weaken. Exercise can help keep the joints healthy and strong.

4. Poor posture

Poor posture can lead to joint pain, as it can put extra stress on the joints. It can also affect the alignment of the spine, leading to back pain.

5. Diet

Diet can also play a role in joint pain. Consuming a diet high in sugar and processed foods can lead to inflammation, which can contribute to joint pain. A diet high in fruits, vegetables, whole grains, and lean proteins can help reduce inflammation and improve overall joint health.

6. Smoking

Smoking can also contribute to joint pain. It can cause damage to the cartilage and other tissues in the joints, leading to pain and stiffness. Smoking can also affect circulation, which can make it harder for the body to heal from injuries.

Other causes

1. Bursitis

Bursitis is a condition that occurs when the bursae, small fluid-filled sacs that cushion the joints, become inflamed. This can cause joint pain, stiffness, and swelling.

2. Tendinitis

Tendinitis is a condition that occurs when a tendon, the tissue that connects muscles to bones, becomes inflamed. It can cause joint pain, stiffness, and limited mobility.

3. Osteoporosis

Osteoporosis is a condition that causes the bones to become weak and brittle. It can increase the risk of fractures and joint pain.

Infections

Infections can also cause joint pain. They can occur in the joints themselves, or in other parts of the body and spread to the joints. Infections can cause inflammation, which can lead to joint pain, swelling, and stiffness.

Joint pain can be caused by various factors, including medical conditions, injuries, and lifestyle factors. It is important to identify the underlying cause of joint pain in order to develop an effective treatment plan. Treatment may include medications, physical therapy, lifestyle changes, and other interventions. It is also important to maintain overall joint health through regular exercise, a healthy diet, and other lifestyle factors. If you are experiencing joint pain, it is important to talk to your healthcare provider to determine the cause and appropriate treatment. We'd be looking at all of that in the next chapter.

CHAPTER 2

TRADITIONAL TREATMENT

1. Ayurveda

Ayurveda is an ancient Indian system of medicine that uses natural remedies to treat a range of ailments, including joint pain. Ayurvedic treatments for joint pain are based on the principle of balancing the three doshas – Vata, Pitta, and Kapha – which are believed to govern the body's overall health and wellbeing. Ayurvedic treatments for joint pain may include:

Massage: Ayurvedic massage techniques such as Abhyanga, Shirodhara, and Pinda Sweda can help to reduce inflammation and relieve pain in the joints.

Herbal remedies: Ayurvedic practitioners often prescribe herbal remedies for joint pain, such as turmeric, ginger, ashwagandha, and boswellia. These herbs have anti-inflammatory properties and can help to reduce pain and stiffness in the joints.

Yoga: Yoga is a form of exercise that has been practiced in India for thousands of years. It can help to improve joint flexibility and reduce pain and stiffness in the joints. Specific yoga postures such as Trikonasana, Vrikshasana, and Virabhadrasana can be especially beneficial for joint pain.

Diet: Ayurvedic practitioners may recommend specific dietary changes to reduce joint pain. For example, they may suggest consuming more anti-inflammatory foods such as fruits, vegetables, whole grains, and legumes while avoiding foods that can exacerbate inflammation, such as processed foods, sugar, and saturated fats.

2. Acupuncture

Acupuncture is an ancient Chinese therapy that involves the insertion of fine needles into specific points on the body to stimulate the body's natural healing processes. Acupuncture has been used to treat a range of conditions, including joint pain. The needles used in acupuncture are very thin and are inserted into the skin at specific points, which correspond to different parts of the body.

Acupuncture is believed to work by stimulating the body's natural pain-relieving mechanisms and promoting the flow of energy (Qi) through the body. It can help to reduce inflammation, relieve pain, and improve joint mobility. Acupuncture is often used in conjunction with other traditional treatments for joint pain, such as herbal remedies and massage.

3. Chiropractic

Chiropractic is a form of alternative medicine that focuses on the diagnosis and treatment of musculoskeletal disorders, particularly those affecting the spine. Chiropractors use manual manipulation of the spine and other joints in the body to improve joint function and reduce pain and stiffness.

Chiropractic treatments for joint pain may include:

Spinal manipulation: Chiropractors use their hands or a small instrument to apply a controlled force to the joints in the spine, which can help to improve joint function and reduce pain.

Soft tissue therapy: Chiropractors may use massage or other soft tissue techniques to reduce muscle tension and improve joint mobility.

Exercise: Chiropractors may prescribe specific exercises to improve joint strength and flexibility.

Dietary advice: Chiropractors may offer dietary advice to reduce inflammation and improve joint health.

4. Traditional Chinese Medicine

Traditional Chinese Medicine (TCM) is an ancient system of medicine that has been used in China for thousands of years. TCM treatments for joint pain are based on the principle of balancing the body's energy (Qi) and restoring harmony to the body's systems

CHAPTER 3

THE NATURAL WAY

1. Turmeric

Turmeric is a spice commonly used in Indian and Middle Eastern cuisine. It contains a compound called curcumin, which has anti-inflammatory and antioxidant properties. Studies have shown that curcumin may help reduce joint pain and stiffness in people with osteoarthritis and rheumatoid arthritis.

One study published in the Journal of Medicinal Food found that a turmeric extract was as effective as ibuprofen in reducing pain and improving function in patients with knee osteoarthritis. Another study published in the Journal of Alternative and Complementary Medicine found that curcumin was more effective than a placebo in reducing joint pain and swelling in patients with rheumatoid arthritis.

To incorporate turmeric into your diet, you can add it to curries, stir-fries, smoothies, or teas. You can also take turmeric supplements, but be sure to talk to your doctor first if you are taking any medications or have a history of gallbladder problems.

2. Ginger

Ginger is another spice with anti-inflammatory properties that may help reduce joint pain. It contains compounds called gingerols and shogaols that have been shown to have analgesic effects.

A study published in the Journal of Medicinal Food found that ginger extract reduced pain and stiffness in patients with osteoarthritis of the knee. Another study published in the International Journal of Rheumatic Diseases found that ginger capsules reduced joint pain and inflammation in patients with rheumatoid arthritis.

To incorporate ginger into your diet, you can add it to teas, smoothies, or stir-fries. You can also take ginger supplements, but be sure to talk to your doctor first if you are taking any medications or have a history of gallbladder problems.

3. Omega-3 Fatty Acids

Omega-3 fatty acids are essential fatty acids that are found in oily fish such as salmon, mackerel, and sardines. They have anti-inflammatory properties that may help reduce joint pain and stiffness.

A study published in the Journal of the American College of Nutrition found that omega-3 supplements reduced joint pain and stiffness in patients with rheumatoid arthritis. Another study published in the Journal of Nutrition found that omega-3 supplements reduced joint pain and stiffness in patients with osteoarthritis of the knee.

To incorporate omega-3 fatty acids into your diet, you can eat oily fish or take fish oil supplements. Be sure to talk to your doctor first if you are taking any medications or have a history of fish allergies.

4. Capsaicin

Capsaicin is a compound found in chili peppers that has analgesic properties. It works by reducing the amount of substance P, a neurotransmitter that transmits pain signals to the brain.

A study published in the Journal of Pain found that capsaicin cream reduced joint pain and stiffness in patients with osteoarthritis of the hand. Another study published in the Journal of Rheumatology found that capsaicin cream reduced joint pain in patients with rheumatoid arthritis.

To use capsaicin, you can apply capsaicin cream to the affected area. Be sure to follow the instructions on the label and avoid getting it on your eyes or mucous membranes.

5. Epsom Salt

Epsom salt is a type of magnesium sulfate that is commonly used in bath salts and foot soaks. It Is believed to help reduce inflammation and pain in joints by promoting relaxation and improving blood circulation.

A study published in the Journal of Evidence-Based Complementary and Alternative Medicine found that soaking in an Epsom salt bath helped reduce pain and stiffness in patients with osteoarthritis.

To use Epsom salt, you can add it to a warm bath and soak for 20-30 minutes. You can also create a foot soak by adding Epsom salt to a basin of warm water and soaking your feet for 20-30 minutes.

6. Massage

Massage is a natural remedy that can help reduce joint pain by improving blood circulation, promoting relaxation, and reducing muscle tension.

A study published in the Journal of Bodywork and Movement Therapies found that massage therapy improved joint mobility and reduced pain in patients with osteoarthritis of the knee. Another study published in the Journal of Alternative and Complementary Medicine found that massage therapy improved joint mobility and reduced pain in patients with rheumatoid arthritis.

To receive a massage, you can visit a licensed massage therapist or learn self-massage techniques to use at home. Be sure to talk to your doctor first if you have any underlying health conditions or injuries that may be worsened by massage.

7. Exercise

Exercise is an important natural remedy for joint pain as it helps improve joint flexibility, strength, and range of motion. Low-impact exercises such as walking, swimming, and cycling are recommended for people with joint pain as they are less likely to cause further damage to joints.

A study published in the Journal of Clinical Rheumatology found that exercise improved joint pain, stiffness, and function in patients with osteoarthritis. Another study published in the Journal of Rheumatology found that exercise improved joint function and quality of life in patients with rheumatoid arthritis.

To incorporate exercise into your routine, start with gentle activities such as walking or swimming and gradually increase intensity and duration. Be sure to talk to your doctor first if you have any underlying health conditions or injuries that may be worsened by exercise.

8. Heat and Cold Therapy

Heat and cold therapy are natural remedies that can help reduce joint pain by improving blood circulation, reducing inflammation, and promoting relaxation.

A study published in the Journal of Physical Therapy Science found that heat therapy improved joint range of motion and reduced pain in patients with knee osteoarthritis. Another study published in the Journal of Rheumatology found that cold therapy reduced joint pain and stiffness in patients with rheumatoid arthritis.

To use heat therapy, you can apply a warm compress or take a warm bath or shower. To use cold therapy, you can apply a cold compress or ice pack to the affected area.

In conclusion, natural remedies for joint pain can provide relief and improve joint health. Turmeric, ginger, omega-3 fatty acids, capsaicin, Epsom salt, massage, exercise, and heat and cold therapy are all natural remedies that can help reduce joint pain and stiffness. It is important to talk to your doctor before trying any natural remedies, especially if you are taking any medications or

have any underlying health conditions

CHAPTER 4

HERBS

- Turmeric

Turmeric is a spice that has been used for centuries in traditional Ayurvedic medicine. It contains a compound called curcumin, which has been shown to have anti-inflammatory properties. Inflammation is a common cause of joint pain, so it makes sense that turmeric might be effective in managing joint pain.

Several studies have looked at the effectiveness of turmeric in reducing joint pain. One study found that turmeric extract was effective in reducing pain and improving function in people with osteoarthritis of the knee. Another study found that a combination of turmeric and ginger was more effective than a placebo in reducing knee pain.

Turmeric is generally considered safe when taken in small doses, but larger doses may cause stomach upset. It may also interact with certain medications, so it's important to talk to your doctor before taking turmeric supplements.

- Ginger

Ginger is a root that has been used for medicinal purposes for centuries. It contains compounds called gingerols and shogaols, which have anti-inflammatory properties. Like turmeric, ginger may be effective in reducing joint pain.

Several studies have looked at the effectiveness of ginger in reducing joint pain. One study found that ginger extract was effective in reducing pain and improving function in people with osteoarthritis of the knee. Another study found that a combination of turmeric and ginger was more effective than a placebo in reducing knee pain.

Ginger is generally considered safe when taken in small doses, but larger doses may cause stomach upset. It may also interact with certain medications, so it's important to talk to your doctor before taking ginger supplements.

- Boswellia

Boswellia, also known as frankincense, is a resin extracted from the Boswellia serrata tree. It has been used for centuries in traditional Ayurvedic medicine to treat inflammatory conditions. Boswellia contains compounds called boswellic acids, which have anti-inflammatory properties.

Several studies have looked at the effectiveness of boswellia in reducing joint pain. One study found that a combination of boswellia and turmeric was effective in reducing pain and improving function in people with osteoarthritis of the knee. Another study found that boswellia was effective in reducing pain and improving function in people with osteoarthritis of the knee.

Boswellia is generally considered safe when taken in recommended doses, but it may interact with certain medications, so it's important to talk to your doctor before taking boswellia supplements.

● Willow Bark

Willow bark is the bark of the willow tree. It contains a compound called salicin, which is similar to aspirin. Salicin has anti-inflammatory and pain-relieving properties, which makes willow bark an effective natural remedy for joint pain.

Several studies have looked at the effectiveness of willow bark in reducing joint pain. One study found that willow bark extract was effective in reducing pain and improving function in people with osteoarthritis of the knee. Another study found that willow bark was effective in reducing pain in people with low back pain.

Willow bark is generally considered safe when taken in recommended doses, but it may interact with certain medications, so it's important to talk to your doctor before taking willow bark supplements.

- Glucosamine and Chondroitin

Glucosamine and chondroitin are supplements commonly used to treat joint pain. They are both natural compounds found in cartilage, which is the tissue that cushions the joints.

Several studies have looked at the effectiveness of glucosamine and chondroitin in reducing joint pain. One study found that a combination of glucosamine and chondroitin was effective in reducing pain and improving function in people with osteoarthritis of the knee. Another study found that glucosamine was effective in reducing pain in people with osteoarthritis of the knee.

While these supplements are generally considered safe, some people may experience side effects such as stomach upset or allergic reactions. They may also interact with certain medications, so it's important to talk to your doctor before taking glucosamine and chondroitin supplements.

- Omega-3 Fatty Acids

Omega-3 fatty acids are essential fatty acids found in fatty fish such as salmon and tuna, as well as in supplements such as fish oil. Omega-3 fatty acids have anti-inflammatory properties, which makes them effective in reducing joint pain.

Several studies have looked at the effectiveness of omega-3 fatty acids in reducing joint pain. One study found that fish oil supplements were effective in reducing joint pain and stiffness in people with rheumatoid arthritis. Another study found that omega-3 fatty acids were effective in reducing joint pain and stiffness in people with osteoarthritis of the knee.

Omega-3 fatty acids are generally considered safe when taken in recommended doses, but they may interact with certain medications, so it's important to talk to your doctor before taking omega-3 supplements.

- SAMe

SAMe, or S-adenosylmethionine, is a natural compound found in the body that plays a role in many biological processes, including the formation of cartilage. SAMe supplements have been shown to have anti-inflammatory properties, which makes them effective in reducing joint pain.

Several studies have looked at the effectiveness of SAMe in reducing joint pain. One study found that SAMe was effective in reducing pain and improving function in people with osteoarthritis of the knee. Another study found that SAMe was effective in reducing pain in people with fibromyalgia.

SAMe is generally considered safe when taken in recommended doses, but it may interact with certain medications, so it's important to talk to your doctor before taking SAMe supplements.

● Devil's Claw

Devil's claw is a plant native to southern Africa. It has been used for centuries in traditional medicine to treat inflammatory conditions such as joint pain. Devil's claw contains compounds called iridoid glycosides, which have anti-inflammatory properties.

Several studies have looked at the effectiveness of devil's claw in reducing joint pain. One study found that devil's claw was effective in reducing pain and improving function in people with osteoarthritis of the knee. Another study found that devil's claw was effective in reducing pain in people with low back pain.

Devil's claw is generally considered safe when taken in recommended doses, but it may interact with certain medications, so it's important to talk to your doctor before taking devil's claw supplements.

Herbs and supplements can be an effective natural remedy for joint pain. However, it's important to talk to your doctor before taking any supplements, as they may interact with certain medications. Additionally, it's important to take supplements in recommended doses to avoid any potential side effects. While these natural remedies can be effective in reducing joint pain, they should be used in conjunction with other treatment options, such as exercise and physical therapy, for best results.

CHAPTER 5

DIET & LIFESTYLE

Dietary Changes

1. Anti-inflammatory foods: Inflammation is a major cause of joint pain, and certain foods can exacerbate it. Conversely, there are foods that have anti-inflammatory properties that can help reduce joint pain. These foods include fatty fish (such as salmon, tuna, and sardines), nuts (such as almonds and walnuts), fruits

(such as strawberries and blueberries), vegetables (such as spinach and kale), and spices (such as turmeric and ginger). Incorporating these foods into your diet can help reduce inflammation and joint pain.

2. Omega-3 fatty acids: Omega-3 fatty acids are essential fatty acids that have anti-inflammatory properties. They can be found in fatty fish, flaxseed, chia seeds, and walnuts. Incorporating these foods into your diet can help reduce inflammation and joint pain.

3. Vitamin D: Vitamin D is important for bone health, and a deficiency in this vitamin can lead to joint pain. Vitamin D can be found in fatty fish, egg yolks, and fortified dairy products. It can also be obtained through exposure to sunlight. If you are not getting enough vitamin D through your diet or sunlight, consider taking a vitamin D supplement.

4. Antioxidants: Antioxidants are compounds that can help reduce inflammation and protect the body from damage caused by free radicals.

Foods that are high in antioxidants include berries, dark chocolate, and green tea. Incorporating these foods into your diet can help reduce inflammation and joint pain.

5. Calcium and magnesium: Calcium and magnesium are important minerals for bone health, and a deficiency in either of these minerals can lead to joint pain. Calcium can be found in dairy products, leafy greens, and fortified foods. Magnesium can be found in nuts, seeds, and whole grains.

Lifestyle Changes

- Exercise: Regular exercise is important for maintaining joint health and reducing joint pain. Exercise can help improve joint flexibility and strength, reduce inflammation, and promote weight loss, which can alleviate pressure on the joints. Low-impact exercises such as swimming, cycling, and yoga are particularly beneficial for people with joint pain.

- Weight management: Maintaining a healthy weight is important for reducing joint pain, particularly in weight-bearing joints such as the hips, knees, and ankles. Losing even a small amount of weight can help reduce joint pain and improve joint function.

- Stress management: Stress can exacerbate joint pain, so it is important to manage stress effectively. Activities such as meditation, deep breathing, and yoga can help reduce stress and promote relaxation.

- Joint protection: Protecting your joints from injury is important for reducing joint pain. This may involve using proper posture, wearing supportive shoes, and avoiding activities that put excessive stress on the joints.

- Rest and recovery: Rest and recovery are important for allowing the body to heal and reduce joint pain. If you are experiencing joint pain, it is important to take breaks and rest when needed. Additionally, getting enough sleep is important for promoting healing and reducing inflammation.

CONCLUSION

Joint pain can be a frustrating and debilitating condition, but there are several diet and lifestyle changes that can help reduce pain and improve joint health. Incorporating anti-inflammatory foods, omega-3 fatty acids, vitamin D, antioxidants, and calcium and magnesium into your diet can help reduce inflammation and promote bone health. Regular exercise, weight management, stress management, joint protection, and rest and recovery are all important lifestyle changes for reducing joint pain. If you are experiencing joint pain, it is Important to consult with your healthcare provider to rule out any underlying medical conditions and to develop a comprehensive treatment plan.

In addition to these diet and lifestyle changes, there are also several other treatment options for joint pain, including over-the-counter or prescription pain medication, physical therapy, and joint injections. Your healthcare provider can help determine the best treatment options for you based on the cause and severity of your joint pain.

It is also important to note that certain lifestyle habits can exacerbate joint pain. Smoking, for example, can increase inflammation and contribute to joint pain. Additionally, excessive alcohol consumption can lead to nutritional deficiencies and contribute to joint pain.

Making dietary and lifestyle changes can be an effective way to reduce joint pain and improve joint health. Incorporating anti-inflammatory foods, omega-3 fatty acids, vitamin D, antioxidants, and calcium and magnesium into your diet can help reduce inflammation and promote bone health. Regular exercise, weight management, stress management, joint protection, and rest and recovery are all important lifestyle changes for reducing joint pain. Consult with your healthcare provider to develop a comprehensive treatment plan for your joint pain

Natural remedies for joint pain are effective and safe alternatives to conventional treatments. The use of herbs, supplements, and lifestyle changes can help to manage joint pain and improve joint health without the side effects associated with prescription medications.

One of the key takeaways from this book is that natural remedies can be used as part of a comprehensive approach to joint pain management. A combination of natural remedies, such as exercise, dietary changes, and stress reduction techniques, can help to reduce inflammation, improve joint mobility, and alleviate pain.

Herbs and supplements have been used for centuries to manage joint pain, and many of them have been scientifically studied and proven to be effective. Turmeric, ginger, and boswellia are examples of herbs that have anti-inflammatory properties and can help to reduce joint pain. Supplements like glucosamine and chondroitin have been shown to improve joint function and reduce pain in individuals with osteoarthritis.

In addition to herbs and supplements, lifestyle changes such as exercise and dietary modifications can also be effective in managing joint pain. Regular exercise can help to strengthen the muscles and improve joint mobility, while a healthy diet that includes anti-inflammatory foods can help to reduce inflammation in the body and promote joint health.

Stress reduction techniques, such as meditation and yoga, can also be beneficial in managing joint pain. Stress can contribute to inflammation in the body, and learning how to manage stress can help to reduce the overall level of inflammation and alleviate joint pain.

It is important to note that natural remedies are not a cure for joint pain. While they can help to manage symptoms and improve joint health, they may not be able to reverse damage that has already been done to the joints. It is important to consult with a healthcare provider before beginning any new natural remedies, especially if you are taking medications or have a medical condition.

Overall, natural remedies for joint pain offer a safe and effective alternative to conventional treatments. By incorporating herbs, supplements, and lifestyle changes into your daily routine, you can manage joint pain and improve joint health without the side effects associated with prescription medications.